new

THE LAYMAN'S GUIDE TO FOOT AND HEEL PAIN

∧

79 570 059 6

<u>Contact Dr Les Bailey</u>

The Clinic (branches across the UK)

Tel – 0845 520 1950

Email – Drlesbailey@yahoo.co.uk

www.thecliniconline.co.uk

The *new* Layman's Guide to Foot and Heel Pain

Les Bailey, Ph. D.

MILTON KEYNES LIBRARIES

DON | 10|10

617.585 BAI

NOTE:

The contents of this book are exclusively from
past/current clinical findings of Les Bailey, PhD.,
and do not reflect the policy or procedures of any
current, past or future clinic or companies at
which Dr Bailey may practise.

Copyright © Les Bailey, PhD., 2005

The right of Les Bailey to be identified
as the author of this work has been asserted by him in
accordance with the Copyright, Designs
and Patents Act 1988.

First published 2005
Revised edition 2006
Reprinted 2006, 2008
Third edition 2009
Reprinted 2010

ISBN : 978-095621-300-6

All rights reserved.
No part of this publication may be reproduced or
transmitted in any form or by any means, electronic
or mechanical, including photocopy, recording or any
information storage and retrieval system, without
permission in writing from the publisher.

Printed through SS Media Ltd - www.ss-media.co.uk

CONTENTS

DEDICATED TO

My tens of thousands of past patients - my warmest regards to you all.

To my children Luke, Connie, Grace and Henry, and my lovely grandson, John - I love you all.

To the memory of Peter Bell, my original "teacher" in orthotics – thanks mate – rest in peace.

To my sister, Christine –
a wonderful sister and a brilliant office superstar!

To Michael Nightingale, who taught and helped me through osteopathic college.

To the academic staff of OIUCM - thank you for trawling through my 10,000-word PhD thesis. Not an easy task!

And finally to my mum 'Kitty', and to the memory of my dad, Les Bailey Snr. You are greatly missed.

PREFACE TO THE THIRD EDITION

I'm absolutely amazed! This book has sold around 25,000 copies in the first and second editions and a further 3,000 in this third edition!

Reviews and kind words on the book's content have been overwhelming, and multitudes of patients have come to see me at clinics as a result of their having read the book, and we are sure that can only mean fewer people suffering from foot or heel pain and better able to enjoy their lives.

I sincerely thank you for reading the book, and I or another of our biomechanics consultants look forward to helping you.

Sending you my heartfelt thanks, kind regards and best wishes for the future.

Les Bailey, PhD.
July 2010

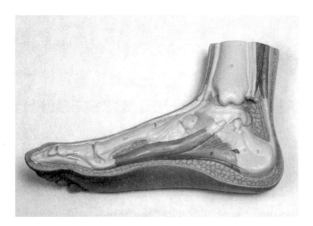

Normal foot

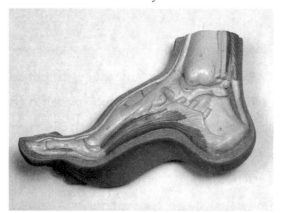

Pes cavus

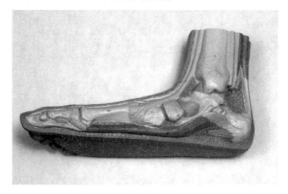

Pes planus

INTRODUCTION

I am passionate about feet! They are a miracle, an engineering marvel not even seen by the likes of Ferrari or Rolls Royce. My original training was as an osteopath, but as soon as I began dealing and specialising in biomechanics I was hooked. The way the foot works is wonderful to say the least. I sincerely hope you enjoy reading this book and that in some way those beautifully designed and created vehicles on the ends of your legs will benefit from your having soaked up a little knowledge from this humble volume.

"Allo, Allo, Allo!"

Many years in our distant past, there existed an ailment known to the population at large as "policeman's heel" (perhaps policeman's "hell" may have described it better) which was said to strike those who walk all day. Policemen used to pound on their regular beat (a rare sight nowadays) and this is where the nickname emanated from.

There were also sore feet, bad arches, and aching feet at the end of the day. One can imagine folk sat around their radiograms, feet soaking in hot water, with a glass of gin

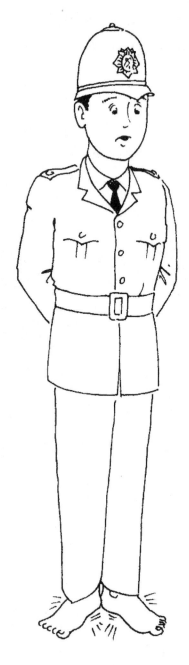

"Policeman's" heel

and a pipe full of tobacco. Some of these people who were "in the know" would purchase metal shoe inserts and just perhaps, if very lucky, gain a little relief. Others would take aspirin to relieve the symptoms while a great deal of the population would have consulted a physiotherapist for a dose of the latest electro-medical treatment. Ah, the bad old days . . .

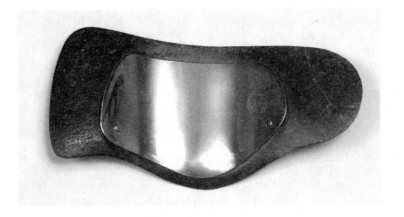

An old-fashioned metal orthotic (!)

But now ...

In the 21st Century things have progressed somewhat. We have a medical name for policeman's heel, which is *plantar fasciitis*, known to cause heel and arch pain in many unfortunate people. People sit round their computer games or widescreen TVs, their feet swathed in ice or rested on a hot water bottle. Some people go to the local chemists and buy one of many off-the-shelf insoles, which, if they are very lucky, may give a little pain control. Some ladies or gents opt for a visit to the doctor to be given anti-inflammatories or a locally stabbed hydrocortisone injection, which generally either misses the pain site or only affords a few weeks scant relief. Many find themselves in the physiotherapist's room having a new improved electro-medical device strapped to their painful feet. Whilst others of a New Age persuasion may choose *chi* energy crystals or organic wholemeal reflexology!

So what's new, Pussycat?

Excuse us for being so bold as to enquire, but what on earth has actually changed? The above, past and present, illustrate the fact that not a lot has actually altered over the passing of time, and symptomatic treatment is still the norm.

Whilst the medical profession has become incredibly adept at saving lives, curing diseases that were life-threatening 50 years ago and bringing forth some amazingly skilled doctors and surgeons, it has done very little to effectively rid the population at large of biomechanical foot pain. Many operations have emerged for the conditions suffered by the feet, occasionally effective, but most with great risk, very little result, or even the chance of more pain as a post-operative prospect.

The understanding of foot pain amongst all branches of medicine is poor to say the least. GPs have very little time to understand it. Most have surgeries bursting at the seams and patients with far greater and more dangerous diseases to be concerned with. A GP's life is not an easy one, and with the constant stream of time-wasters they encounter, how would they ever get the time to specialise in foot pain? The same can be said of orthopaedic surgeons. The old and outdated operation of removing the spur has ceased. In some cases operations are carried out to release the *aponeurosis* (the support under your arch which connects the heel to the metatarsals) but luckily this is rare and carries with it the high risk of failure or exacerbation of pain.

The general concept of *plantar fasciitis*, in its many guises, is poorly understood by all branches of the medical profession: physiotherapists, osteopaths, chiropractors and podiatrists all seem to miss the vital point that *plantar fasciitis* is a very individual complaint, each case being unique. Every case of foot pain and biomechanical misalignment has a root cause and each person is unique in their needs.

Most practitioners treat *plantar fasciitis* or metatarsal pain as a nuisance complaint rather than the painful, crippling problem it really is.

Our aim is true

The aim of this book is to enlighten the lay person and hopefully to stimulate further research by students and practitioners in all branches of medicine.

Even from the viewpoint of my own original training as an osteopath, a so-called "complete" learning in musculoskeletal medicine, our course covered little about heel and foot pain. The foot as a subject was hurriedly brushed over. We seek to open the eyes of the man or woman in the street to the causes and treatments for what can only be described as a severely debilitating group of conditions.

"No-one understands!"

Do our medical practitioners have any concept of how the patient feels, with every footstep marred by dull or sharp pain to the heels, arches or metatarsals? Not just one specific move, but every step? The private practitioner who gladly takes money for short-lived temporary relief has surely never lived with the pain of those first few steps every morning. The GP books you in to a physio-therapist who uses ultrasound and gives you stretching exercises but all to no avail. I sometimes wonder if these practitioners have any idea of the pain felt by the patient and the abject misery it causes.

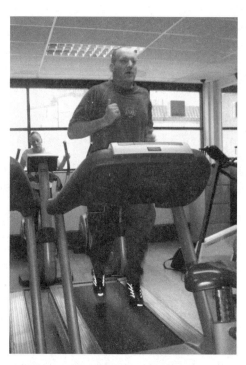

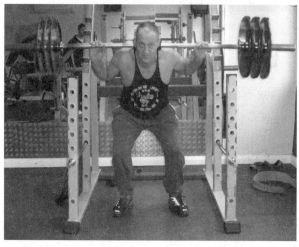

The author can now run and lift heavy weights on his feet despite having once had severe plantar fasciitis

Me? Dramatic?

Perhaps I sound a little dramatic, as not all cases are absolutely excruciating. But from my side of the fence, I have specialised in dealing with some of the most difficult cases of foot pain. We see all age-groups, from young children to the very elderly, some early or mild cases and some presenting on crutches. The one thing the longer standing cases have in common is that they have tried every medical discipline before arriving on our doorstep. They generally feel they have been "through the mill" of the medical profession, both complementary and mainstream. Patients are shocked when we locate the causative factors of their case and don't try to fob them off with mere pain control. However, as I always tell patients, we do have the luxury of specialising exclusively in our field.

It is my belief that in order to best empathise with a condition, a practitioner should first have experienced it; so I shall tell my own story of how I stumbled into my specialisation.

"Run, Forrest, run!"

I was first introduced to heel pain some 22 years ago. It reared its ugly head while I was pounding the pavements on my twice daily seven mile runs. Being a Thai boxing fighter, these runs were a necessity to maintain peak aerobic fitness and despite always running in proper running shoes, it soon became mighty obvious that the biomechanical faults in my feet were to play havoc. Not only was I experiencing heel pain, but my shin splints were getting worse by the week. To many readers, the first signs I felt will sound familiar. I thought I had trodden on a stone. My heel felt bruised and my arch felt strained and painful.

"Don't run, Forrest, don't run!"

The next few weeks saw the symptoms go from bad to worse. I employed all the usual things people try, such as ice packs, anti-inflammatories, heat, massage, ultrasound; all to no avail. Eventually I saw a friend of mine who was an orthopaedic sports specialist, a doctor who spent his career treating sporting injuries.

He treated my shin splints with hydrocortisone, a grossly painful and ridiculous procedure considering what my later research into biomechanical medicine would bring to light. He diagnosed *plantar fasciitis* with a heel spur growth (and automatically blamed the harmless spur) which was confirmed on X-ray. This showed that the problem was not a new one and that my running, although it had forced the problem to the surface, had not been the sole causative factor. Both my parents suffered *plantar fasciitis* in later life, so the cause was highly likely genetically poor foot posture. He had a podiatrist prescribe me some rigid orthotics which were made using a plaster cast. He then injected hydrocortisone into the area locally which hurt like mad. Neither had much effect.

My shin splints and heel pain were back with a vengeance. I was even having to use swimming as a cardiovascular exercise as I could no longer run. Even walking, whilst not as severe as I would witness in patients in later years, was a displeasure. I tried all sorts of off-the-shelf orthotics, pads and gels from chemists and finally used some so-called orthotics from a high street foot specialist. Their staff chiropodist prescribed me some orthotic devices which caused a bruised feeling to pervade the entire foot. They were at a complete loss as to how to adjust them and demonstrated no biomechanical knowledge whatsoever.

A very lucky meeting

It was purely by chance that I attended an osteopathic conference - something I rarely did, because I found it hard to stay awake throughout dull and uninteresting lectures. One of the trade exhibitors at the conference was a man named Peter Bell, who, little did I realise, was about to change my entire life and start me on a journey to the realms of biomechanical medicine. In short, Peter led me by the nose into my specialised field. He had on display some new types of orthotics from the USA. We got talking and I told him of the problems I had personally experienced both with heel pain and shin splints. I told him how I had tried different orthotics, which brought forth a look of amusement from Peter. After further talking I decided not to attend the next lecture, and stayed with Peter for the rest of the day. He took his own particular type of cast from my feet and arranged that my orthotics would be with me in a few weeks.

For the rest of the day Peter waxed lyrical about the specialist materials used in their prescription orthotics from the USA and how Britain was still using outdated methods of manufacture and poorly designed materials. His zest and enthusiasm got to me, and looking back, my interest in osteopathy took a downturn in favour of working with foot biomechanics.

Eureka!

Three weeks later my orthotics arrived, fresh from the land of Uncle Sam, and I wondered whether they really would solve my problems. On day one I inserted them, and at first they felt fine. Two hours later I could quite happily have discarded them. My arches hurt like mad, but I was advised to persevere. By day two things were getting easier and by day three all pain had gone. Over the next few weeks the pain in my heels disappeared, the shin pain had abated and I was able to return to my heavy running and training schedule, pain-free. Four minor adjustments were made to the orthotics and I was back to normal. As "easy" as that, it seemed.

Peter guided me through much post-graduate training, plus his own personal tuition. My life's vocation was just beginning.

I began prescribing orthotics from my clinic in Buckinghamshire, where, through reputation only, I went from prescribing two or three pairs a month to being inundated with painful feet from all around the area. The conditions I was treating ranged from heel pain to knee problems, ankle instability, sacroiliac pain and all manner of biomechanical problems. The success we had even in those early days astounded me.

That was a far cry from the clinics I have worked in across the UK, where patients arrive from all over the country and abroad and where we prescribe the orthotics using a 3D optical foot laser linked to our specialist laboratory in the USA.

Enjoy this book and take heart. If I and thousands of others can be helped, I feel sure you will.

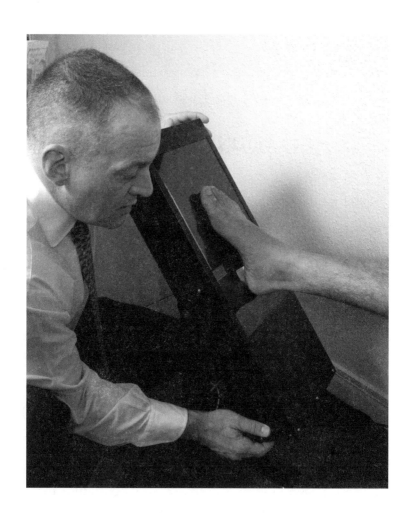

A 3D optical laser foot scanner - a useful measuring device.

"PIONEERING"

How I developed our unique orthotic system

The phenomenal success rate I enjoy with our orthotic system did not come about by accident. Our cure rate went from 20% to over 90% by applying a lot of thought and experimentation to not only the foot shape but to its **function.**

I have seen every type of orthotic ever produced, all brought into consultations by patients looking for a permanent solution. They all ask me why the orthotics they have been prescribed, or have been bought for them, have not worked. Thankfully, this is easy to explain.

I have seen orthotics that range from the most expensive "Harley Street" type to the blatantly ridiculous "gimmick" type purchased from the internet. I have taken a handful of these to explain why they simply cannot work.

"Cheap and cheerful" (Off the shelf)

The major problem with these is that they merely push your feet from one wrong position to another, placing your feet into a "fake" posture. Pardon my scepticism here - but isn't that why the problem occurred in the first place? Going from one wrong posture to another absolutely *cannot* give you the results you need and will very likely push your knees and hips into an unfavourable position.

Prescription orthotics

The prescription orthotics doled out by practitioners all over the world have made little or no technical progress in all the years I have been involved with foot problems. They are still too rigid and can cause irritation and bruising to an already inflamed arch and heel, as well as preventing natural movement in the foot structure.

Conversely, we see many "soft pads" passed off as orthotics and these may, if you're lucky, mask the pain temporarily.

My early pioneering work

The work with *plantar fasciitis* and general foot pain (for which I eventually received my doctorate) began with simply putting some thought into what was going wrong with prescription orthotics and why these were getting very poor results with *plantar fasciitis* and metatarsal pain.

I first looked at this some 15 years ago and realised that many aspects of the foot's function were being overlooked.

I noticed where the mistakes were (and indeed still are!) being made and that nobody was thinking past foot <u>shape</u> alone. Foot shape alone is very easy to capture with a prescription orthotic and can be correctly achieved by using laser, plaster cast or even a foam cast. Yet orthotics are still being made too rigid or too soft to allow any kind of proper solution to *plantar fasciitis* or metatarsal pain.

I decided to "pioneer" a system whereby the foot can be reshaped and allowed to function <u>correctly</u>.

This was not an easy task and it took the skill of some very advanced technicians to realise my ideas. It involved much experimentation with patient weight, height and foot type along with their chosen footwear. However, we now have a phenomenal success rate and tens of thousands of happy patients as the fruits of our labour and as a practitioner, as well as a pioneer, this was very pleasing.

So many crazy ideas

I have borne witness to some crazy ideas put forward and still used in the world of orthotics. I will list a few here and the reasons why I consider them hopeless.

Our feet must first be in a position known as "talar neutral" to lose all excessive muscle, bone and ligament strain, and this involves the feet being measured in their non-weight-bearing state to capture this position.

There is a so-called laser/computer method of measurement that is used extensively. This requires the patient to stand on a pressure pad to be measured, thus capturing the feet in their faulty posture, the exact same stance that has caused the symptoms in the first place!

I have seen patients' feet strapped into "night splints" overnight, pulling the feet taut. This merely prevents the micro-tearing from healing and, to my mind, causes worse tearing than before.

I see clinics now employing the same 3D optical foot lasers we use, but using these to supply rigid standard orthotics, which merely irritate the foot.

My general observation over much clinical time has seen a new "craze" emerge at least once a year to treat *plantar fasciitis*, each claiming to be the Holy Grail. I have stuck to my original pioneering work and just seen our results get better and better. Put simply, the only way to treat these difficult cases is to return the feet to their correct position <u>and</u> function. Without this, any treatment used to speed healing, except in a low percentage of cases, cannot work. Full stop.

Common treatments for foot and heel pain and why they fail

- **Cortisone injections**

Let me say from the outset, I am not totally opposed to the use of cortisone. I use it for certain sports injuries and, where the area can be allowed to rest, it can be wonderful. Arnica injections given locally come under the same listing.

However, in foot pain cases, its use long-term is pointless. It can only give temporary relief, because until the foot posture and function are corrected, the cause of the problem is still there.

Cortisone *can* be useful in cases where healing is slow even with correct orthotics, but this is rarely needed except in cases where the medial fascia (inner foot) is concerned.

This can be notoriously slow to heal, so a little help can be useful, and cortisone or arnica are two ways to stimulate healing.

- **Anti-inflammatories/pain killers**

Nearly every patient who has ever consulted me has been prescribed anti-inflammatories by their GP. I have no issue with this as some cases that may have an injurious onset can benefit from this approach. Examples could be perhaps a jumping/landing injury causing an acute (short-lived) episode to the arch or heel. Another possibility is that of the keen DIY enthusiast, possibly painting a ceiling and standing constantly on the balls of the feet upon a ladder. This may give rise to a strain injury to the arch and/or heel.

However, any *plantar fasciitis* case where the symptoms are present for more than approximately three weeks has the very real danger of turning into a chronic (long-term) case. In these cases anti-inflammatories or pain killers are positively hazardous, because when the symptoms are hidden by drug therapy the patient feels able to do more activity than the injured foot can bear, thus leading to further injury long-term.

• **Physiotherapy/osteopathy/chiropractic/acupuncture**

All these use various approaches and may employ ultrasound, laser therapy, deep tissue massage, acupuncture, manipulation, etc.

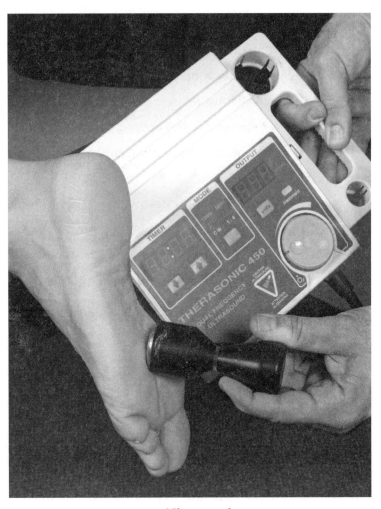

Ultrasound

All of these disciplines, excepting the more "wacky"
ones, are brilliant in their own right for a legion of
problems but in *plantar fasciitis* or metatarsal pain, all you
will achieve is the equivalent of an expensive pain killer -
in short, temporary relief. No treatment can hope to

remove the biomechanical *cause* of *plantar fasciitis* or metatarsal pain, including even such "revolutionary" treatments as short-wave therapy or similar.

But (and there is always a 'but') these can be extremely useful where the patient has proper orthotics and faster healing is wanted, or the individual patient is slow to heal, as certain people are.

- **Local arnica injections**

Around 20 years ago, I acquired some injectable homoeopathic arnica which I used after Thai boxing injuries. It was very useful as a systemic treatment, meaning I injected it under the skin in much the same way a diabetic would inject insulin. The effect was to assist the whole body to heal from injury far quicker (I found arnica tablets ineffective on me personally).

My naturally enquiring mind wondered if anyone had ever used this locally in the same way hydrocortisone is used, at the site of tears or soft tissue injuries. I assumed it would have been used like this before and began to trawl the internet, books and records. To my utter amazement, nobody had even thought of it.

I was not going to experiment on anyone else before myself, so I waited until I had an injury.

Some weeks later, whilst out road-running, I slipped on a divot and caused a three-ligament tear to my ankle. I limped home realising this injury could take 6 weeks minimum to heal and tentatively injected arnica directly into and around the ligaments and rested directly afterward. To my amazement I was able to run again, pain-free, the very next morning.

I began to experiment on fellow Muay Thai fighters (knowing arnica had no real side effects) and the success rate came back at around 60%, which I believe, from observation, is the same as hydrocortisone. Feeling very encouraged by this I contacted a private doctor who did his own trials and we are now able to use this effectively on patients who have had orthotics to greatly assist healing.

Given its inherent safety, I was rather pleased with myself for having pioneered this and I hope doctors or surgeons reading this will be encouraged to make their own trials. Spread the word, so that more patients can benefit !

Note to practitioners/doctors/surgeons

Injectable homoeopathic arnica is available from "Weleda".

I generally use 6 x potency for acute cases and 30c for chronic cases. Please contact me and let me know your thoughts and findings. I feel this mode of treatment has enormous potential in many areas of musculoskeletal and even dental cases and hope that in the future many may benefit from it.

Stretching exercises/night splints

This is a treatment method which must be approached with very great caution. The foot displaying *plantar fasciitis or* metatarsal pain is already suffering tearing and inflammation along the *plantar aponeurosis* (the support under the arch which connects the heel to the metatarsals) which can be greatly irritated and worsened by these senseless exercises.

If you must use stretching exercises, wait until the *plantar fascia* is healed and then use them for general prevention only. You have been warned!

• Night splints

My favourite gripe is another form of "stretching" named the "night splint".

This device, which resembles something from a medieval torture-chamber, stretches the foot upward at night, holding the tears in the plantar aponeurosis open. This means they cannot heal, so that when you step out of bed in the morning, no pain is felt.

The reason for this is simple: our bodies carry out natural healing whilst we sleep, and the tears go through their first stage of this, namely the forming of adhesions.

Upon rising in the morning these re-tear and hurt! A night splint merely prevents this first healing stage from occurring, which is, frankly, idiotic. This is a prime example of 'no pain, no gain'.

- **Operative procedures**

Let's get one thing straight. I admire surgeons greatly. They are amazingly clever and dedicated people whose skills save millions of lives every year and whose brilliant work deserves a lot more recognition for service to humanity than it receives.

However, I see very poor results in surgery cases for *plantar fasciitis* and metatarsal pain, except in the very rare cases where rigidity is such a powerfully overwhelming factor that even orthotics cannot solve it without surgical intervention (and even then orthotics are still needed post-operatively to prevent further new tearing and foot collapse).

Let us take a layman's look at the various surgical procedures currently available.

Surgery for the treatment of *plantar fasciitis* remains controversial - I have seen many failures and some exacerbations, but I have also seen some successful cases where surgery has definitely worked. However, I question whether the risk of this surgery could have been avoided if the correct orthotics had been used, as in my own practice I have probably sent only 10 people for surgery in over 20 years!

Generally, the surgical procedure will go as follows:

An incision is made along the heel then the medial calcaneal nerve is located and checked. In rare cases this nerve may be released should it be entrapped. The medial 30-50% of the fascia is released (cut) at its origin.

If a spur is present it is generally removed (almost always needlessly!)

Muscles are then divided to release the nerve, if this is entrapped.

The wound is then closed by stitching and the patient is put into a cast and kept completely non-weight-bearing for at least 3 weeks.

After healing, an orthotic must be prescribed to avoid further biomechanical causative factors.

Endoscopic plantar fascia release is also being carried out with somewhat more success.

Problems with surgery

Complications arising from this surgery can include numbness, neuroma formation and, obviously, further pain. Fractures can result from spur excision and problems often result from arch instability causing overload at the heel and metatarsals, resulting in stress fractures. Additionally, there are the usual post-operative difficulties of wound infections and healing crisis.

My own advice is to regard surgery as an absolute last resort - and I know the surgeons themselves would recommend the same approach.

"First-flush" *plantar fasciitis*
Stamp on early *plantar fasciitis* (but not literally!)

We see many, many cases of *plantar fasciitis* where the history is of a mild or early attack some years, months or weeks previously which then "disappears".

Be warned - it is far more prudent to catch *plantar fasciitis* at its 'first-flush' stage and to thus prevent the major attack that will surely follow. Even if first-flush has been and gone, orthotics will be a very wise precaution which will hopefully prevent an otherwise inevitable further attack.

In short, never ignore even a brief episode of *plantar fasciitis*.

CHAPTER ONE

INSPIRATION FOR THE SUFFERER

We realise, from many years in our field and from hearing horror stories from our patients, that countless people go down every avenue in search of a cure for their pain, and most become very cynical. This cynicism is perfectly understandable, as knowledge in the field of *plantar fasciitis* is poor to say the least. However, we would like to inject a little sunshine into your life regarding the whole ghastly affair, with some inspirational cases that have been treated using very specialised orthotics.

Case one: 40 years of suffering!

Although we have treated many cases where people have suffered for ten, twenty or even thirty years, my favourite "long termer" was the prison officer who had lived with *plantar fasciitis* for 40 years. His employment necessitated him having to walk on stone floors for eight hours or more every day. I cannot begin to imagine the exacerbation of pain caused by this constant pounding on hard, unforgiving concrete, day in, day out. We diagnosed the cause, which was mainly pronation causing a constant pulling on the *plantar fascia*, causing it to become rigidised, semi-flexible. Orthotics were prescribed to correct this pronation, and he opted for a little manual treatment from our remedial therapist to hurry the healing along a little. Two days after receiving the orthotics he strolled into the clinic wearing a smile usually kept in reserve by showbiz personalities and ... you've guessed it. . . pain free.

We must emphasise that not all cases go as quickly as this but, thank God, most respond quite rapidly.

Case 2 - A bet?

In 2002 a lady in her early thirties, consulted us in considerable pain. She had been prescribed rigid orthotics made from a plaster cast by a local podiatrist. Upon examination, we found that they had exacerbated the symptoms by literally bruising the *plantar fascia* and had thrown the feet into excessive supination. She was very satisfied with what I told her, so we assessed the correct orthotics and set about laser scanning her feet. The next day her father rang me, absolutely fuming that she had spent money on what he considered was exactly what she already had. I explained why I had replaced what she had, but he was difficult to placate. After further conversation it transpired we were members of the same gentlemen's club. A friendly bet was wagered that if I was wrong I would refund his daughter and buy him dinner at the club. He still owes me dinner!

Case 3 - Marathon man

Mr G., a man in his late 40s, sporting a pair of NHS crutches, arrived at our clinic quite unable to walk unaided. He had been a keen runner but had been afflicted by severe *plantar fasciitis* for three years, and he had used the crutches for the past six months. Upon examination he presented with very high arches *(pes cavus)* and rigid, unforgiving feet. We used orthotics to "bridge" the high arch, which is a procedure requiring great accuracy. The result, four months later, was a gentleman who was in training for the London Marathon.

Acres of diamonds

We see our successes as acres of diamonds; thousands of happy people able to walk again, pain free. I realise that when you have been in pain for a long time and had your hopes raised and dashed many times in search of a cure, it is all too easy to give up. The best advice I can give is to start from the beginning again. Mentally erase all you have been told about your condition and re-evaluate it.

Or, as the psychologists would say, do a paradigm shift in your mind and learn to cast a new light on the challenge at hand.

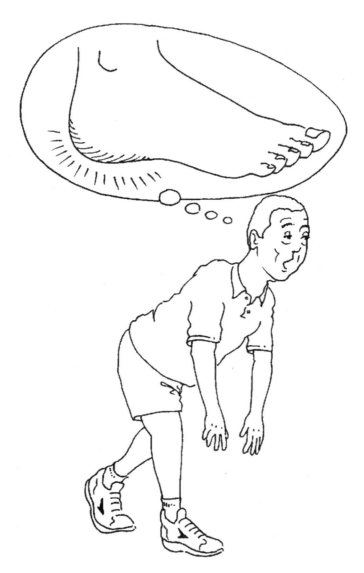

Sometimes it's all you can think of

CHAPTER TWO

THE PSYCHOLOGY OF FOOT PAIN

Those readers suffering from heel and foot pain will know only too well the abject misery of constant pain and how debilitating it can be, not only physically but mentally too. The things you used to take for granted such as playing football or tennis, or going on a long walk with your partner, all cause pain with every step taken. Even a walk round the shops on a Saturday is a battle of wills between you and your feet, which even the best retail therapy will not cure.

The search for those magic shoes that will clear the problem goes on and on and you live in trainers as that is what you have been told is best. You can't go out with your partner to social functions that require you to dance or stand up and, what's more, your partner is beginning to feel the strain of your bad feet too.

In desperation you try every kind of practitioner but nothing works. Depression, and a general lack of faith in the medical profession, set in. You begin to feel low. Most practitioners tell you that it will go away soon and treat your case like a minor nuisance with as much relevance as a blackhead. To the sufferer, it is a blight on an otherwise great life.

My message is this ... If you are a practitioner, remember, this problem is painful and debilitating. If you can't help, you owe it to your patient to refer them to someone who can. With the greatest of respect, do not treat this condition like it's a minor problem - please! Should you have never experienced *plantar fasciitis* at its worst, place some marbles in your shoes at the area of the arch. Now bang the middle of the heel five or six times with a hammer and start walking immediately. After five minutes' walking, remove the marbles and walk again. That, my friend, is how your patient feels.

This lack of understanding often extends to family, friends and colleagues. You should try to understand that they cannot see *plantar fasciitis*. The feet are, curiously, one of those areas of the body that are never discussed in polite society. The general public's attitude toward sex, religion, race and all the old taboos may have softened almost to a point of acquiescence . . . but *feet*? Oh, not in front of the Vicar!

Now all of this is made worse by many people assuming that because they cannot see your foot pain, that you are simply becoming lazy. One of the most common complaints we hear from patients is how much weight they have gained due to their painful feet. To put it bluntly, as we all know, inactivity piles on the pounds. Inactivity is also bad for the heart and circulation. Not good.

At last...

It is always a pleasure to see our new patients in the waiting room reading the numerous thank you letters on display. Former patients write these as a testimonial to how grateful they are. The look on the new patient's face is one of raised hope and a feeling of "at last".

In 2002, the Daily Mirror wrote a full page article on the work which one of my past clinics did with *plantar fasciitis*. The response was nothing short of astounding. Just a few seconds elapsed between people phoning and requesting appointments. This carried on for days and we were kept busy for months afterwards. I mention this here simply because the thing that struck me so forcibly was the sheer desperation in people's voices and the relief they expressed afterwards. It was as though they had found a drinking fountain in a desert.

Let's get positive

It has been proven time and time again that the patient's mental attitude plays a major part in healing. Before you undertake to rid yourself of foot pain (or any disease), you must get your brain into a positive mode. Just making do with a life spent in pain is not enough. Your hopelessness and frustration lead to a depressed, angry state that can result in giving up on ever finding a cure. You can become apathetic and just 'switch off'. The truth is that you have to employ massive action to get your active life back again!

Start by setting a goal in your mind and put down on paper the steps you want to take from this book to get you back to full function again. For example you may want to start with hot and cold packs, a wobble board, or even the ultimate step towards correct orthotics. Give yourself a timescale for each and actually write down your intentions. This will feel so powerful and positive as it puts you in charge of the journey to a cure. The mental capacity and power inside you as a human being is so much more awesome than you know. Please - don't just sit back and accept this problem. Begin the great mental fight.

As the great sportswear manufacturers Nike said: "Just do it".

No failures

When treatment after treatment fails to yield results, remember, it's not the end of the world. You or the practitioner have not failed. You have merely discovered another way that doesn't work for you. Now you can go on to the next method. Never give up hope. Refuse to accept any negative thoughts that you will not recover from these problems and go, go, go! You *will* recover and today is the first day of your new journey to a cure.

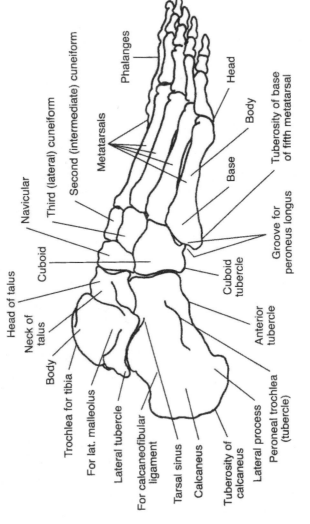

Head of talus

Neck of talus

Navicular

Third (lateral) cuneiform

Second (intermediate) cuneiform

Phalanges

Metatarsals

Head

Cuboid

Body

Base

Tuberosity of base of fifth metatarsal

Groove for peroneus longus

Cuboid tubercle

Anterior tubercle

Body

Trochlea for tibia

For lat. malleolus

Lateral tubercle

For calcaneofibular ligament

Tarsal sinus

Calcaneus

Tuberosity of calcaneus

Lateral process

Peroneal trochlea (tubercle)

Lateral view

- 46 -

CHAPTER THREE

RELEVANT ANATOMY

I have called this chapter relevant anatomy, as I have no intention of boring the lay reader with irrelevant anatomical studies that bear no relation to what they need to know in order to gain a better understanding of their own feet.

The human foot combines an amazing mechanical complexity with structural strength which is able to hold your body weight superbly. The ankle and foot serves as a foundation, shock absorber and propulsion engine, sustaining enormous pressure, particularly whilst running or jumping.

It contains 26 bones - one quarter of the body's total. There are 33 joints and over 100 muscles, tendons and ligaments. These are nourished by a huge network of blood vessels, nerves, skin and soft tissue.

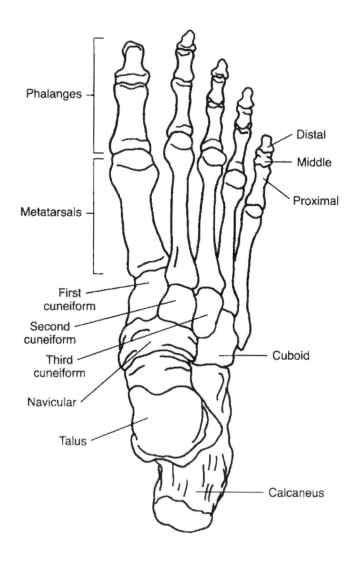

Phalanges

Distal
Middle
Proximal

Metatarsals

First
cuneiform
Second
cuneiform
Third
cuneiform
Navicular
Talus

Cuboid

Calcaneus

This little piggy...

In anatomical terms, the foot is divided into three parts: the forefoot (front part), midfoot (middle section) and hindfoot (the rear part). The forefoot is home to the five toes (phalanges) and their connecting long bones (metatarsals). Each toe is made up of several small bones. The big toe (hallux) has two joints (interphalangeal joints) and two tiny sesamoid bones that enable it to move up and down. The other four toes have three bones and two joints. The phalanges are connected to the metatarsals by five metatarsal phalangeal joints at the ball of the foot. The forefoot bears half the body's weight and balances pressure on the ball of the foot.

The midfoot has five irregularly shaped tarsal bones which form the foot's arch and this serves as a shock absorber. The bones of the midfoot are connected to the forefoot and hindfoot by both muscles and the *plantar fascia*.

The hindfoot is composed of three joints, and links the midfoot to the ankle (talus). The top of the talus is connected to the two long bones of the lower leg forming a hinge that allows the foot to move up and down. The heel bone (calcaneus) is the largest bone in the foot. It joins the talus to form the subtalar joint which enables the foot to rotate at the ankle. The bottom of this large heel

Area for attachment of the deltoid ligament

Medial tubercle of talus

Trochlea for tibia

Groove for flexor halluicis longus tendon

Head and neck of talus

Calcaneus

Medial process

Navicular

Sustentaculum tali

Tuberosity of navicular

Metatarsals

First (medial) cuneiform

Phalanges

Medial sesamoid

Medial view

bone, or "calcaneus", is cushioned from impact by a layer of fat.

A network of muscles, tendons and ligaments supports the bones and joints in the foot. There are twenty muscles in the foot that give it its shape by literally holding the bones in position and these contract and expand to impact movement. The major muscles in the foot are:-

- The anterior tibial which enables the foot to move upward.
- The posterior tibial.
- The peroneal tibial which controls movement on the outer ankle.
- The extensors which help the ankle raise the toes to initiate the act of stepping forward.
- The flexors which stabilise the toes against the ground.

Smaller muscles enable the toes to lift and curl. There are elastic tendons in the foot that connect muscles to bone and joints. The largest and strongest of these is the Achilles tendon, which extends from the calf muscle to the heel. Its strength and function facilitate walking, running and jumping.

Ligaments are like the guy ropes on a circus tent and stabilise and hold everything in place. The longest of these, although not strictly speaking "ligaments", are the *plantar fascia*. This is our major focus of interest.

What is the *Plantar Fascia*?

The *plantar fascia* and *aponeurosis* have a complicated and confusing "press" in many textbooks, which generally either mix everything up or over-complicate the issues.

The *plantar fascia* is composed of fibrous bands of connective tissue. It originates from the plantar medial tubercle of the calcaneum. It is made up of three distinct bands, the medial, central and lateral (1). This explains why some patients experience *plantar fasciitis* pain not only in the middle section of the arch but often in the medial aspects of the fascia, particularly in the area where the medial arch of the foot meets the heel. Occasionally, albeit in fairly rare cases, the *lateral fascia* experiences symptoms too.

Most textbooks are very confused as to the terms and differences in *plantar fascia* and *plantar aponeurosis*. Students are also often confused as to how it is made up - some call it muscle, some refer to it as tendon and some ligament. I feel it is more accurate to term it fibrous bands of connective tissue (1). The reason nature designed it like this is that muscle or tendon alone could not deal with the massive tensile strength that runs through the fascia with every step you take.

It all contains a high number of ligamentous cells which add greatly to its strength

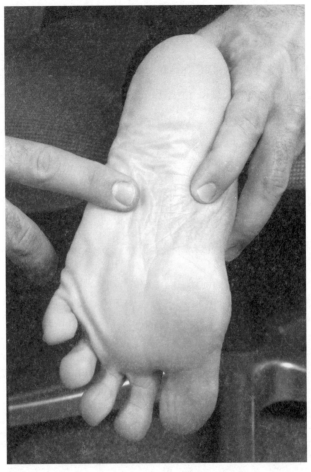

The plantar aponeurosis exposed on the surface

For a more complete anatomical look at the foot and the various layers of the musculature and ligamentous structures of the plantar aspect of the foot, further study would be required outside of the scope of this book. For example see references (2) and (3).

The *plantar fascia* can be considered a major tensile support network of the foot, as it provides maximum support throughout the complicated gait cycle and, as I've already stated, it holds up the arch of the foot during some extremes of weight bearing. These large forces are transmitted between the hindfoot and forefoot during the stance phase of gait (4).

The plantar aponeurosis connects like a tie-beam and forms the longitudinal arch of the foot. It extends from the tuber calcanei to the ball of the foot where it attaches itself with fibres into the skin and the proximal phalanges of the toes (1).

Some sources state that the *plantar fascia* is non-elastic in that it possesses no stretch ability (5) but when diagnosing we have found different types of rigidity by palpation concurrent with different pain patterns, seriousness of symptoms and whether *pes cavus* or *pes planus*. In a nutshell, what I am saying is that not all *plantar fascia* exhibits the same rigidity (or lack of it).

Simply, this is why I have never prescribed a "standard" prescription orthotic! Every patient is different!

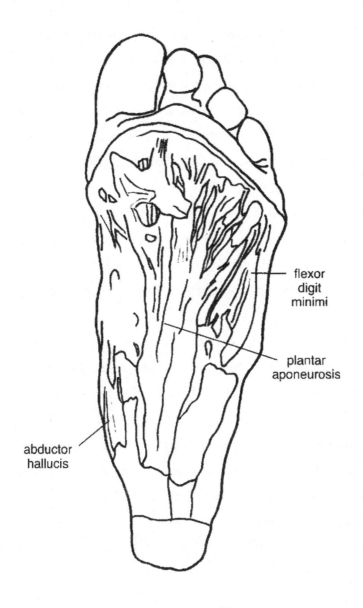

flexor
digit
minimi

plantar
aponeurosis

abductor
hallucis

Underside of foot

Other sources claim that rigidity of the *plantar fascia* comes about with age. Dr William Rossi says, (and I am in full agreement): "the ageing theory is highly debatable"

(6), pointing out that shoeless people of advanced years rarely ever show a loss of foot elasticity.

We find, upon palpation, no age differentiation in cases where the fibres that make up the *plantar fascia* show increased hardness or rigidity.

So we have now looked at the nuts and bolts of how the foot is constructed - the basic anatomy. I hope you may now be stimulated to explore this subject further and to read the books and websites available. The foot is a truly amazing structure and one that, even after having spent so many years working with them, I never tire of their many nuances and problems. For example, imagine how this anatomical miracle a few inches in length supports the body's weight. What is more, the feet propel the body into a walk, jog, run or sprint perfectly, time after time. The feet accept their signals from the brain then set themselves in motion, creating a beautiful synergy between nerves, muscles, tendons, bones and ligaments, to carry an entire human being's weight, wherever its owner cares to take it. Truly amazing.

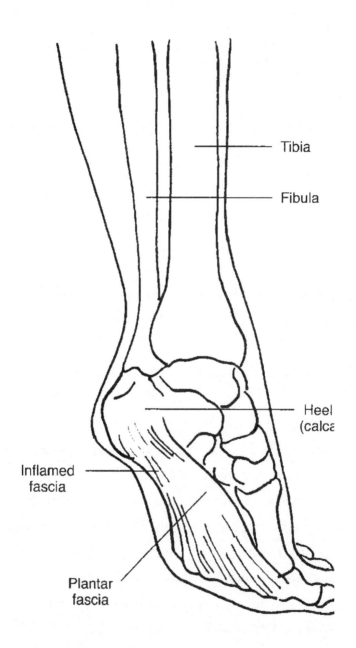

Tibia

Fibula

Heel
(calca

Inflamed
fascia

Plantar
fascia

CHAPTER FOUR

SO WHAT IS *PLANTAR FASCIITIS* OR "HEEL SPUR"?

In simple terms, *plantar fasciitis* is a condition where the *plantar aponeurosis* and/or lateral and *medial plantar fascia* have become overstretched, and perhaps a multitude of micro-tears have occurred throughout their length and possibly even slightly torn away from the heel. This tearing, occurring at the calcaneum, is often called "a spur". However, a true heel spur very rarely causes actual pain, and a high percentage of people walk around with heel spurs who have never had *plantar fasciitis* and who will never have a day's pain. An actual "heel spur" is merely a calcium growth. This has been proved to be painless, and even occurs in people who have never or will never experience pain. The sharp heel pain arises at the point of actual tear of the *plantar aponeurosis* at the *calcaneum*. This may not be torn, but it can be badly inflamed. Some patients experience pain on the medial fascia at the point where the inner area of the arch meets the heel. In short, *plantar fasciitis* takes many forms, and a correct diagnosis as to your own individual cause should always be sought.

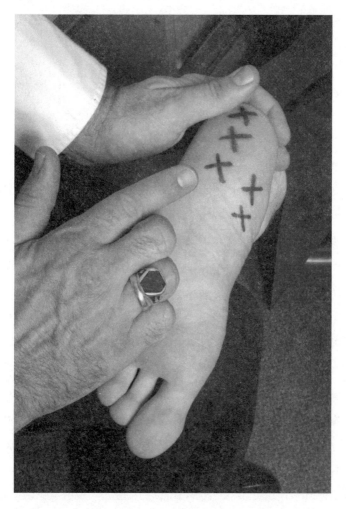

X marks the spot. Sites where heel pain can strike

A genetic cause?

It seems to be common practice in the world of psychology to blame our parents for all our physical or emotional weaknesses. From my own vast experience and observations, many of our foot problems really are genetic, and we gain our foot type from our parents and forefathers. Before you book yourself into counselling to discover if your parents are the root cause of your foot problems, allow me to explain my own personal findings relating to the ancestral link.

I am in the fortunate position of seeing many families presenting in my consulting room; often brothers, sisters and parents. Very often a number of relatives have the same problem, but the main point to make concerning *plantar fasciitis* and its genetic connection is that although the tendency toward getting it is very often inherited, it still takes a particular activity to bring it the fore. A good example of this is that my own parents both had *plantar fasciitis* which began in their sixties, which I was obviously able to clear - like myself, they are both pronators. Yet my own started in my twenties and was brought about by excessive running. The point here is that the link to pronation and p*lantar fasciitis* is very clearly a family weakness. I had "awoken" (as

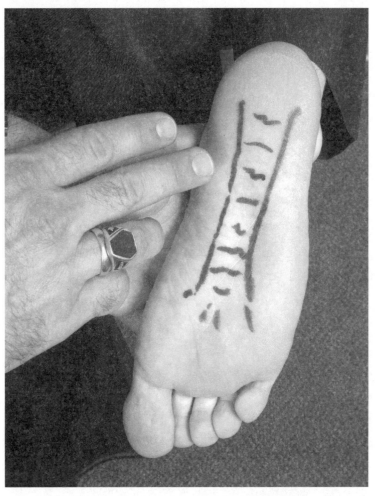

The route of the pain along the aponeurosis

opposed to caused) my own *plantar fasciitis* by a heavy running schedule.

My own findings have been that around eighty per cent of people had exactly the same foot structure as their same sex parent and same sex siblings. Ten per cent showed the same foot structure as their opposite sex parent, and ten per cent had no similarity to either parent. Not all of the parent and sibling matches suffered the same symptoms, but very often just the same intrinsic foot structure e.g. flat feet or high arches. Very often there would be a history of the same heel problems in grandparents and patients will often tell tales of grandfather or grandmother hobbling around after rising from their bed. However, from what I have seen, the problem begins earlier in each generation. (It would be wonderful if a practitioner based in a university had time to prepare official statistics on the above phenomenon.)

Age-related

A question frequently asked by people middle-aged and older is whether *plantar fasciitis* is caused by age. The age link is actually of little relevance, except that, in particular patients, the ligaments supporting the ankles weaken over the years causing a slow and prolonged drop to the medial arch and rearfoot, therefore exacerbating any existing pronation and placing an increased strain on the *plantar aponeurosis*. This minor consideration apart, let us explore the reasons why different age groups may become susceptible to *plantar fasciitis*. I must stress that these are not set in stone, and this is only a general overview.

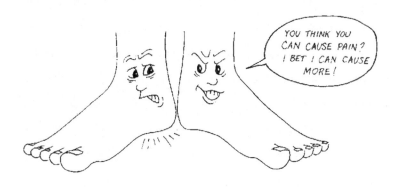

Plantar fasciitis rarely stays in one foot before progressing on to the other

Childhood cases

It is often assumed that all childhood heel or foot pain is brought about by Sever's Disease. A big surprise to many practitioners is that children, as well as adults, do get *plantar fasciitis*. It would appear obvious that deterioration to the elasticity of the *plantar aponeurosis* is not a cause at this age. Our diagnostic eye will immediately turn towards a faulty biomechanical foot posture, such as excessive pronation or cavus. One finds the child is generally of the hypermobile body type; in other words all the ligaments of the body "overstretch" and in the case of the feet, a pronation occurs as a result. A rarer cause we occasionally see is where the child has been born with a rigid and unmalleable *plantar aponeurosis* that will allow no elastic movement during the gait cycle and merely presents with a series of micro-tears along the aponeurosis length. We see this type in people of all ages, but it will generally present itself in children where the child is particularly active, for example in weight-bearing sports.

My own opinion on the connection with Sever's Disease is one which I have not heard expressed by any other practitioner, but which I consider to be anatomically very viable, and which I believe is supported by my numerous successes in this area.

In cases of Sever's Disease, I see the child who has a rigid *plantar aponeurosis* where it connects to the heel. Fractures occur in the bone. My first question is always: "What caused these fractures?" To my mind the exertive pull from the rigid aponeurosis causes the fractures because the bone of a child is not yet fully ossified (hardened).

The role of the orthotic is to stop this pulling effect and regain control on the pull at the heel.

The art of prescribing orthotics to children is not to over-correct the foot to the point where it cannot strengthen during growth. As prescribers, we seek to correct to the point of relieving pressure from the *aponeurosis* by either "bridging" a rigid *aponeurosis* or cavus foot or by supporting a pronator or "flat foot". I suggest that this reinforces my point about not using inaccurate arch lifts (to give just one example). Again I stress, we correct only to this point, and not to the full correction that we would seek to achieve in most adult cases.

I should also add that, having observed many child-hood cases to whom I have given repeat prescriptions over the years, I can say that "Once a pronator, always a pronator". Things do not generally improve, and orthotics will be a desirable prophylactic against biomechanical pattern foot and limb problems for life.

Teenage/early 20s

There is frequently a history of taking part in competitive sports, or of a tough training regime being followed, perhaps into the early 20s. If the reader is inclined to accuse me of blaming the activity for the *plantar fasciitis*, I plead a definite "not guilty". If sporting activity (or any other weight-bearing activity for that matter) had caused the problem, then all sports people would suffer from plantar fasciitis. The message I am trying to convey, and one that I instil into our patients, is that *plantar fasciitis* and other foot problems happen because you are biomechanically susceptible to them. It's as if you are programmed (like a computer) from birth, that one day, out of the blue, one of these problems will occur. All it takes is for you to carry out an activity that will "awaken the sleeping beast". So in effect, the activity is merely an irritating factor and not a directly causative one. I hope this makes the matter clear. If not, with all the greatest respect to the reader, please read the passage again. It is a most important factor in all ages, but is particularly prevalent in young sportspeople. I make no apologies for repeating the above point throughout the book, albeit in different ways, because it is an essential step towards understanding the origins of *plantar fasciitis* and the plethora of biomechanical foot ailments.

Some cases of *plantar fasciitis* in this age group will present simply because they are so pronated, or biomechanically unsound, that the *plantar fascia* and/or *aponeurosis* is under so much stress that the usual problem occurs, with tearing and inflammation throughout.

Middle aged or elderly cases

It is unusual to encounter a *pes cavus* foot presented by a middle aged patient with heel pain. Not unheard of, but unusual. Generally speaking the *pes cavus* subject has had *plantar fasciitis* at a much earlier stage in life.

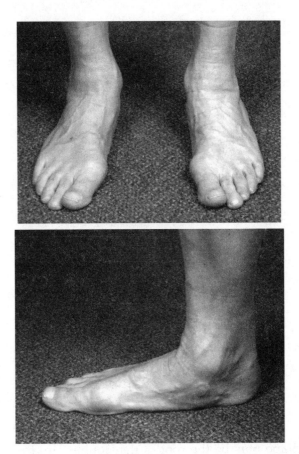

Pronation

The exception here is that, at this age, the ligaments, tendons and connective tissues become more brittle and more likely to tear - the *plantar aponeurosis* being no exception to this - and it is liable to a sudden outbreak of tearing and inflammation at this time of life. This is particularly so with *pes cavus* cases, with their naturally rigid and shorter *plantar fascia*.

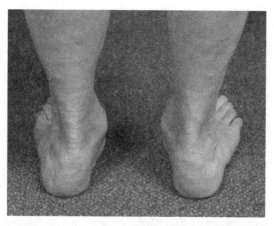

Pronation rear view, noting "bowed" Achilles

The older patients we see tend to be categorised by a number of causative factors. Firstly, it should be understood that there must be an underlying biomechanical reason for the problem. For example, the person will have always been pronated, either midfoot, rearfoot or both or, as we have already stated, a *pes cavus* foot shape may be the root of the trouble. In the case of the pronator, it generally transpires that the pronation is worsening and causing new and more tenacious "pulling" effects on the *plantar aponeurosis*. This further pronation happens because the ligaments holding the foot and ankle stable weaken naturally as we age, but we must resist the temptation to assume *plantar fasciitis* or any other foot problem is merely the result of age as an actual causative factor. With your new knowledge of tangible root causes, I hope the above makes sense to you. Age should more accurately be thought of as an irritating factor, rather than causative.

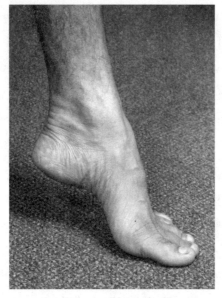

Pes cavus

An interesting consideration ... Asian foot

In our clinic we receive a high number of Asian patients, mainly of Indian origin. The truth is that I have never read or even heard of Asians showing a greater disposition to *plantar fasciitis,* but I shall share with the reader my own unique observations on this matter. I shall not be so arrogant as to claim that this is 100 per cent unique, but I repeat that I have never heard of this being observed before. If any professional readers care to write and correct me I shall happily consider their findings. I am certain that many practitioners of physical medicine have noticed that their Asian patients show a marked propensity toward hypermobility to the musculoskeletal structures. I certainly noticed this in my former work in osteopathy when I treated the entire human framework.

When we look at India through the eyes of an observer of yogic principles, we see it is taught and practised with great relish, and its Indian participants seem to be able to bend into exaggerated positions more easily than their Western counterparts. From this, we begin to see how this hypermobility is a reality. When we observe the anatomical make-up of the *plantar aponeurosis* and its similarity to a ligament, or when we look at the actual ligaments of the foot and ankle, we see how the hypermobility factor irritates the tension of the plantar aponeurosis. I have further observed a phenomenon amongst my Asian patients in that they seem to experience more pain than do other nationalities suffering the same condition. The only conclusion I can reach on this matter is that the ligamentous hypermobility in the ankles must be playing its part by creating a greater tension in the *aponeurosis*, and therefore the heel, than in Western patients. Lifestyle can also aggravate an already existing propensity to the problem (e.g. by standing on hard floors for long periods of time), but again, this does not act as a causative factor but merely as an aggravating one.

CHAPTER FIVE

A LOOK AT EVERYDAY
BIOMECHANICS

Our feet are far from being static structures and correct movement is absolutely essential to the health of the structures of the foot, as well as to the musculoskeletal structures above the foot such as the knees, hips and lower back, even as far as to the temporomandibular joint (jaw), according to some sources. It is the combined and interrelated function of the bones, ligaments, muscles and joints that drives the amazing engineering structures we call our feet to propel the body and enables them to cope with the various walking surfaces we force them to tackle. One of the most complex and poorly understood roles of our feet is in their intrinsically wonderful role of shock absorption.

Any degree of loss of the foot's ability to absorb shock, or an imbalance of shock absorption will lead to faulty weight distribution. This is at the heart of nearly every foot problem. It also explains why drug therapy is rarely, if ever, the answer and why the judicious use of intelligently designed orthotics will most often provide the solution to the problem.

In addition to the natural springiness of the foot's structure, one of its main shock-absorbing features is the heel pad. This layer must play its part by cushioning the foot's impact with the ground.

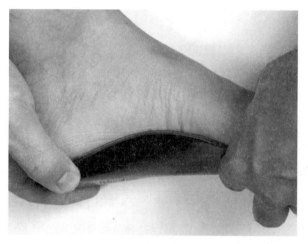

A perfectly fitting arch

We very occasionally use a computerised foot pressure pad at the clinic as part of our diagnostic work. This computerised pad shows where excessive pressure is being exerted when the subject is standing. We generally observe that when a *plantar fasciitis* case stands on the pressure mat, it is on the heels that the main pressure falls, or conversely, at the metatarsal areas in the case of metatarsal pain.

We rarely use this machine, as our clinical experience is beyond this; but it is of interest if only to show biomechanical imbalance in picture form. The completion of the shock absorbing effect is in the eccentric contractions of the foot muscles. Imagine, if you will, the suspension in your car and how this moves each wheel up and down upon uneven surfaces. This is the effect of the eccentric contractions.

The absolutely remarkable work of the foot may be amply illustrated by its innate ability to cope with not only flat surfaces but irregular areas such as the unforgiving "underfoot punishment" of a stony beach, cobble-stoned street or dried bumpy grassland. The foot does this frankly applaudable work by sharing the load between the forefoot, hindfoot, arch and ankle to move, like Byron's poetry, through a sea of natural and counter-balanced motion. The healthy foot glides through these motions neither landing heavily or unevenly, nor firing shockwaves throughout the body.

It is absolutely vital that the foot can cope well with uneven surfaces by showing enough flexibility to, for example, circumnavigate a stone yet remain rigid enough to push-off and propel the body without collapsing at the ankle.

Furthermore, in relation to our friend the plantar aponeurosis, the foot has to display a relaxed form upon standing still, yet be able, without pain, to contract adequately to assist in propelling the body to walk. This fine and dandy balance can only be achieved by a biomechanically healthy foot.

The types of foot affected

There is no one single cause of any type of foot but I would like to simply explain the problems associated with the different types of foot affected. The following is obviously a simplified view and many other diagnostic factors must be added to the equation to extract exact causes and effect a solution.

The most challenging and my personal aesthetic favourite, is the pes cavus foot. This is the proud-looking foot, standing tall and rigid like a stag about to do battle. Its high arch and sloping dorsum surface (upperfoot) give it a sleek appeal resembling the shape of a stiletto shoe.

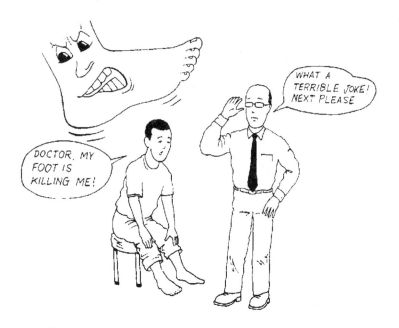

But this is where the svelte and parallel beauty ends. The high arch makes this an unforgiving beast, rigid like an oak tree in a high wind, liable to break. Its *plantar fascia* is like tight, brittle wire, rigid and fibrous. Its other structures and supports follow suit, and this makes them equally unforgiving. This means that the *plantar aponeurosis* is shorter than usual, and almost inevitably acquires either *plantar fasciitis* or metatarsal pain, since all the person's weight is exerted upon the heel and metatarsals, whilst the arch is pulled taut like Robin Hood's bow-string pulling at the insertion in the heel and its joinings at the metatarsal heads. This makes the heel and metatarsal heads behave like two opposing tug o' war teams, ripping at the aponeurosis like weight on a rotten rope.

The pronator or flat foot is the second type for discussion. In this case the inner ankle slumps further inwards as if trying to meet up with its opposite number. It may look as if it were weak through alcohol and unable to bear its own weight; the arches fall flat like deflated balloons. Pronation brings with it many "veritable delights" from the multitude of musculoskeletal shortcomings including ankle pain, shin splints, knee symptoms and certain lower back imbalances.

The major negative issue in the case of *pes planus*, or flat feet, is not only in the resultant stretching of the *plantar fascia* (medial and aponeurosis) but also the heel strike which forces the unfortunate owner of *pes planus* feet to thump across the floor with a thud like a migraine. This has the effect of striking the heels with each step thereby exacerbating the overall problem. Therefore, when prescribing an orthotic in these cases, I always design its effect to absorb heel strike.

The pronator, like the *pes cavus*, is placing constant strain on the *plantar aponeurosis* and fascia by exerting a pull-like effect throughout the entire length. This pulling is caused by the collapsing effect of both ankles and arches pulling the *aponeurosis* away from the heel and pulling at the metatarsal heads. The result of this is micro-tearing and inflammation along the fibres.

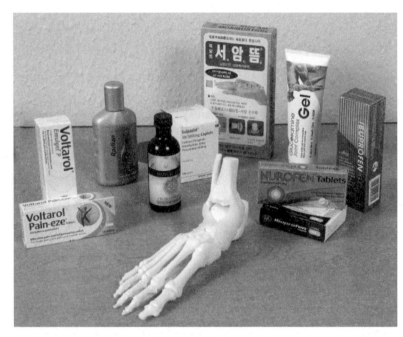

General painkillers

CHAPTER SIX

SELF-HELP FOR HEEL AND ARCH PAIN

It <u>must</u> be remembered that <u>any</u> form of self-help or pain control cannot <u>cure</u> foot pain but may give temporary relief

Self-help is a wide-ranging and very subjective topic, and conjures up images of old ladies mixing up herbal lotions and potions. You may single out or use a mixture of some of the ideas in this chapter. They are not meant as a substitute for professional help as a full and accurate diagnosis should first be sought.

Much of the information given here can be extremely useful to assist in alleviating a certain amount of the pain, and patience and perseverance will be the key.

Hot and cold packs

One of the most powerful anti-inflammatory methods is the hot and cold pack. It rapidly reduces inflammation by pumping fresh blood into the area (hot) and then dissipating it (cold). This literally opens and closes the blood vessels "squeezing" the inflammation away.

For the application of cold I recommend the application of one or more ice-packs - so you will need to keep them lined up in the freezer and constantly available. These can easily be obtained from a chemist or sports shop.

To give you your heat source one may choose a wheat pack that is heated in a microwave, a hot-water bottle or even an infra-red lamp. Heat is heat, whatever the source.

The correct method of application is to place the hot pack on the affected area for five minutes, followed immediately by the cold pack, and repeat as often as you wish or have time for. Try this first for perhaps four times each, as I strongly recommend a 'tester' to ensure you are not one of those rare people who react adversely to this particular treatment.

I would like to share with you an example of how powerful hot and cold packing can be. I remember a case, from when I was practising as an osteopath, which illustrates the remarkable effects that can be achieved by employing this method. A patient consulted me, with his wife in tow. The gentleman was in a terrible state displaying a massive crisis to the sacro iliac joint. They were at great pains to point out that a major financial loss would occur if he were not out of pain in twenty-four hours, or at the very least active enough to carry out the work he had been assigned.

There was severe inflammation and misalignment to the sacro iliac joints which I immediately corrected with osteopathic manipulation, thereby dissipating the cause. However this still left a great deal of inflammation which could have taken days to clear. I told them of the hot and cold treatment and, realising how desperate they were, explained carefully that if they carried out hot and cold treatment for eight to ten hours continuously he should be back on his feet the next day. The credit goes to this man's wonderful wife who painstakingly did a ten-hour shift of constant hot and cold. To rid the area of that much inflammation in such a short time-span demanded little short of a miracle, but his wife's perseverance delivered it.

Shoe padding

In the absence of a proper orthotic you may find shoe padding a useful temporary relief. Please bear in mind the negative effects an off-the-shelf orthotic can have, and do not use any device that is shaped. Avoid, for example, those that have a shaped arch. It is preferable to use a flat bed of sorbothane than can be obtained from a sports shop, or a material with similar shock-absorbing capability. This can act as a useful temporary "padding" and alleviate a little of the pain from the shock of walking.

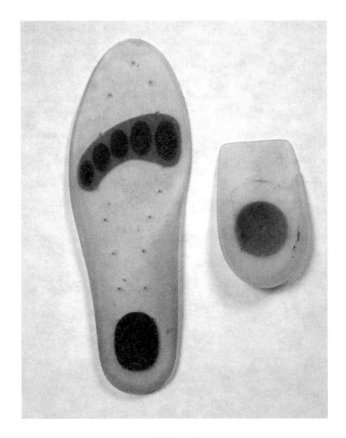

Gel pads

Acupressure

Some people find acupuncture helpful for pain control and you may wish to visit an acupuncturist for this, or try acupressure to acupuncture points at home either using fingertips or a tens machine. Do not over stimulate the points but "coax" them with firm pressure.

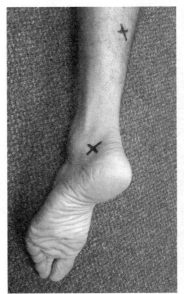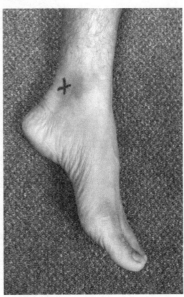

Acupressure points B1 57 and 60 (left) and Ke (right)

The photographs illustrate the points (7) but one may also use "Ah Shi" or local points of tenderness (that is areas directly around or over the pain area that are particularly tender). Stimulate these by fingertips for three to five minutes at each point. You should find that this will have the effect of taking the edge off the pain.

Rest

Obviously extended rest will help with pain; but this is no long-term answer, as no-one wants to live their life in bed or on the couch. Many doctors cite rest as a major healer of foot pain. Unfortunately, they forget that one has to earn a living, and in any case, we have to get up and move at some stage. So as we stand up on badly positioned feet the problem comes flowing straight back.

Changing exercise routines

Many readers will be athletes; they may like to jog or perhaps attend the gym. Pain in the feet, be it from *plantar fasciitis* or any of the numerous other causes can make doing weight-bearing exercises a misery. But with a little willingness we need not lose our fitness, which we can maintain in other ways. If you are a regular runner you may like to substitute a multi-fitness machine or fast swimming. You might prefer to use a bicycle, or a static exercise bike. It is worth noting that exercise keeps our brain and body in peak condition, so we would be wise to avoid abandoning it if at all possible.

Wobble boards

A wobble board is a fine investment and a great self-help method. It is a rare case that I do not prescribe these at the same time as orthotics to assist greater and quicker recovery. A wobble board will quickly strengthen the muscles in the feet and ankles without danger of overstretch to the *plantar aponeurosis*, fascia or Achilles. It works by rapidly strengthening the ankles so that they cease to roll inwards into excessive pronation and thus irritate the *plantar fascia*. You can mimic this effect if you want to demonstrate pronation on the fascia. Simply push your ankles inwards, towards each other, whilst keeping your feet flat on the ground. You will feel a pulling sensation in the arch area. Try to imagine this happening with every step you take. If we can strengthen our ankles we dramatically reduce what is a powerful and destructive irritating factor to the fascia.

The board I choose for patients is fourteen-inches across, and the exercises we favour are shown in the following photographs. Remember that during the early days you may care to hold on to something until your balance has improved. We always advocate wearing shoes when doing wobble board exercises.

I recommend three-to-five minutes twice daily for one month, followed by once daily to maintain ankle strength.

If you wish to make the wobble board a regular thing, it is well worth paying for a lesson from a physiotherapist or researching the internet where you will find some very interesting variations. To buy a wobble board, look to the internet. A wobble board is a very worthwhile investment, and as well as the uses we advocate them for, they are useful for developing balancing skills, as well as toning the legs and bottom area.

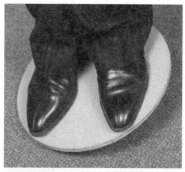

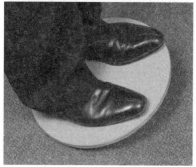

Wobble Board use

Conclusion

Self-help measures can go towards giving you some relief. You will notice I have purposely left out off-the-shelf type orthotics. I believe that these merely push the foot from one faulty position to another and have the potential to create pain and even wear and tear in distant areas of the musculoskeletal system. My strong advice is not even to contemplate sending off for, or buying from chemists or the like, any pre-made orthotic or arch lift.

CHAPTER SEVEN

OTHER CAUSES OF HEEL PAIN

Not all heel pain is attributable to *plantar fasciitis*, although it has to be said it is rare for it not to be. Certain types of heel pain can be associated with forms of rheumatoid arthritis, *ankylosing spondylitis*, and the general rheumatic spectrum of diseases. This goes hand-in-hand with the rheumatic spectrum's inherently inflammatory nature, as well as the general joint laxity that accompanies these diseases. However I will point out that with the correct orthotics I have had astounding success with many cases where rheumatic spectrums were an issue. Not all had one hundred per cent success but many were helped fifty to sixty per cent just by skilfully releasing the strain being put on the *plantar fascia* and Achilles by correcting the individual's gait. Faulty gait coupled with rheumatic spectrum disease processes can lead to joint stress and progressive damage.

There is evidence drawn from some texts that link certain types of heel pain to gout, which is caused by a renal excretory problem in ninety per cent of cases, or over-production of uric acid. The usual site for gout to attack is the hallux (big toe) which presents as hot, red and incredibly tender. In rare cases gout can also affect the subtalar joint, Achilles and heel.

Retrocalcaneal bursitis occurs as a result of irritation to the bursa sac at the back of the heel. It is usually associated with badly fitting shoes. Generally speaking ultrasound, ice and backless shoes worn for a period of time provide the patient with a satisfactory outcome.

Puncture wounds to the heel may cause infection such as *cellulitis, osteomyelitis, osteochrondritis* and *septic arthritis*. A puncture wound can occur where the patient has trodden on a sharp object for example. With infections of this kind, a doctor's advice must be sought.

Direct trauma such as a very high jump or fall onto the heels may give rise to localised fracture at the heel area.

Nerve entrapment of the medial calcaneal nerve elicits pain that travels up the leg and is of a sharp electrical nature. It is thought to be due to excessive pronation of the foot causing micro trauma to the heel.

A dermatome is an area of skin that is fed by a major spinal nerve. Dysfunction of the relevant spinal area will elicit a sensation of numbness and/or pain. The particular dermatome that goes over the heel runs from S1, the first portion of the sacrum. A competent osteopath or chiropractor should be able to carry out relevant tests to determine if a dermatome is the problem.

It must be remembered that the above conditions are relatively rare, and even though we as a clinic specialise in heel and foot pain, we seldom encounter these conditions.

(For information on Sever's Disease see relevant text.)

CHAPTER EIGHT

OTHER COMMON BIOMECHANICAL FOOT PROBLEMS

I am including the following chapter in the hope that it will stimulate further reading. I will not go into great detail on each condition but a little additional understanding can only be helpful. However, always remember that self-diagnosis is never a great idea and the opinion of a competent practitioner should be sought to confirm, or issue, a valid diagnosis.

The recommended reading section at the back of this book will give you some ideas about which books to purchase or borrow from the library, in order to pursue your points of interest further.

There are huge lists of foot conditions which we could outline, showing many rare and very occasionally seen foot problems, but to keep the interest of the layman I shall seek to give a brief outline of conditions we see and treat on a fairly regular basis.

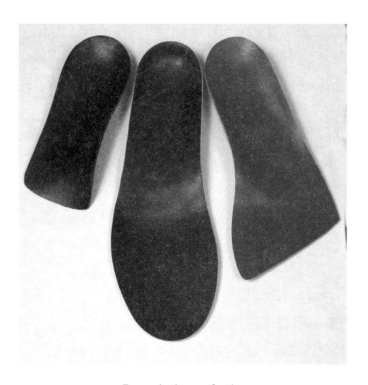

Prescription orthotics

Metatarsal madness (Metatarsal pain).

The most common problem, other than *plantar fasciitis,* that I am called upon to treat is metatarsal pain (the ball of the foot). There are several metatarsal conditions; the first we shall look at is the dropped metatarsal. Generally the practitioner encounters thickened skin over the under surface of the two middle metatarsal heads (the middle section of the ball of the foot). This is where they have been forced downwards out of their natural arch (the metatarsal arch). The skin grows into calluses as a protective shell against the ground strike of these two middle metatarsals. This problem is compounded in people who have very little fat layer to the ball of the foot. When we encounter this, the metatarsals are like bony knobs hiding just under the skin. My question as a diagnostician is: exactly why have these metatarsal heads dropped? Common thought among practitioners is that the ligaments supporting the metatarsal heads merely weaken and allow the dropping effect to occur. I have a major issue with this and always seek to find out why. Generally I will diagnose a problem with the *plantar aponeurosis*, its surrounding tissues, and the unnatural amount of pulling against the metatarsal heads forcing them downward. My own thoughts on this and my clinical findings indicate that metatarsal drop is merely another form of *plantar fasciitis* and indeed in a great majority of cases it does accompany *plantar fasciitis*. It is the normal practice to concentrate on the use of just a metatarsal dome to raise the heads, but my own method is to seek to temper the *plantar aponeurosis* by correctly balancing the strain upon it and getting it to cease pulling at the metatarsals.

If I had a hammer — Hammer Toes

We see a lot of hammer toes during our day-to-day practice. These are due to the metatarsal heads being dropped and the unfortunate results are that the toes "claw" to try to stabilise the forefoot in its ground contact. If these are not tackled very early the tendons are inclined to shorten and even with corrective orthotics the toes need to be straightened either by regular manual manipulation or by surgery in more stubborn examples.

"Me Mortons is killing me Doctor!" – Mortons Neuroma

We see hundreds of cases of this vicious little complaint every year. To put it in a nutshell, it's a growth on the nerve or nerves at the point where they run through the metatarsal heads. These will be diagnosed by a practitioner firstly by carrying out a "squeeze test" to the foot which may elicit a sharp pain at the very area the growth is occurring. Secondly ultrasound scanning can be used when there is any doubt. The approach we take is relative to the individual case. For example we are never content to concede that a Morton's neuroma has occurred for no reason in a perfectly biomechanically sound foot. We usually witness pronation causing a "bunching" to the metatarsal heads meaning that the heads squeeze together. It is my belief that the neuroma forms in order to protect the nerve against pressure exerted by the metatarsal heads, one clashing against the other and literally squeezing the nerve. Therefore the approach which seems to yield the best results is first to use an orthotic with a metatarsal dome to raise and space out the heads so as to relieve the burden of pressure on them. Secondly, by correcting pronation and the medial arch we relieve the bunching pressure to the metatarsal heads. Usually this will solve the problem on its own but sometimes the neuroma has got larger and a simple operation is needed to excise it. The orthotic is now needed more than ever as the neuromas will return or further ones will occur without its prudent use. We see many patients with multiple neuromas where operations have been successfully carried out to remove them but the "cause" has not been tackled and further ones have returned.

"Left, right, left, right" – March Fractures

The next metatarsal problem is the march fracture which chooses the second/third metatarsal heads as its most frequent site. Amongst the cases I have dealt with I have found it incredibly rare for the cause not to be associated with dropped metatarsal heads and sometimes including a distinct lack of fat-padding under the metatarsal heads. It is stated in the usual non-enquiring way that it occurs due to over-use in athletes or in soldiers after route marches. I would question this assumption. Whilst I agree that it happens during these activities, I suggest that as it does not happen to *all* soldiers or *all* athletes then there must be some other intrinsic cause.

"More sugar, Vicar?" – Diabetes and Orthotics

The diabetic foot gives rise to its own problems such as neuropathy (decreased nerve function) or necrosis (circulatory problems associated with blood vessels). People with *diabetes mellitus* have a naturally increased risk of fracture as bone-mass is reduced. Orthotics as part of the diabetics strict foot health regime must firstly be rigid enough to be effective, yet soft enough to avoid the danger of fracture should the person wish to run or do any athletic activity. The softness, particularly in the top cover, is paramount so as not to bruise delicate blood vessels.

It is my belief that orthotics should be a part of all diabetics' (type 1 and 2 {*mellitus* and *insipidus*}) foot-care regime, but these must be properly prescribed as described above.

The tunnel of love – Tarsal Tunnel Syndrome

Tarsal tunnel syndrome is, to all intents and purposes, carpal tunnel syndrome of the foot. The tarsal tunnel is where the major nerves pass through on their journey into the foot. This compression causes burning and sharp pain to the inner ankle and arch area of the foot, sometimes even travelling to the big toe (hallux).

Its causes tend to be either an earlier ankle injury or as the result of a weak collapsing arch which, in turn, increases pressure on the nerve inside of its tunnel.

Tarsal tunnel syndrome <u>must</u> firstly be treated with orthotics to take away the cause. This is absolutely <u>vital</u>.

Secondly, there may be a need to use cortisone to calm the nerve or, in some cases, surgery may be required to complete the cure.

An interesting footnote on tarsal tunnel syndrome that I have observed is that it is very often accompanied by *plantar fasciitis*. This is not surprising as the same causes that elicit tarsal tunnel syndrome can also cause *plantar fasciitis*.

I have often heard surgeons tell patients that orthotics are not the answer, but this is a very short-sighted view, as orthotics must be a major part of its treatment (but not necessarily the <u>only</u> part).

"I think there's a rod in my toe?" – Hallux rigidus

Hallux rigidus or *limitus* are conditions in which it is difficult to bend the stiffened big toe. Put simply the joints in the big toe become arthritic; the two joint surfaces wear away leaving osteophytes and semi-fusing of the joint. Use of orthotics has been shown to aid *hallux rigidus*, especially in its infancy, by taking pressure away from the hallux itself. Should this prove to be of only limited use directly, the toe can be fused surgically which generally proves satisfactory. We have usually found a combination of orthotics and physical therapy such as manual traction to the hallux, heat treatment and soft tissue massage to be extremely useful. Shoes worn must be of a kind which will not permit the toe to compact against the end.

"Ooh, me poor ol' bunions!" - Bunions

Bunions, or more correctly *hallux abductor valgus*, are either caused by a genetic disposition or a combination of pronation coupled with tight shoes. Genetic factors are thought to account for over half of cases. For example this may be due to an ancestral tendency toward pronation or, as some suggest, the inheritance may be a taste for the wrong type of footwear. The role of orthotics is to take the weight away from the big toe joint and relieve it of pressure. We have found this to be extremely effective clinically, and some reduction in the size of the bunion may even occur. Pain will subside and the bunion will not enlarge further. Surgical intervention will be an option for those who desire the hallux straightened for cosmetic reasons, but this should not be undertaken lightly as, like any surgery, there is a possibility that you may be left in pain. On a more positive note, this procedure is usually very effective and really is a case of personal informed choice.

"Who dares shins!" – Shin Splints

Shin splints presents as a pain on the inner (medial) side of the shin bone. It is commonest in runners but can affect

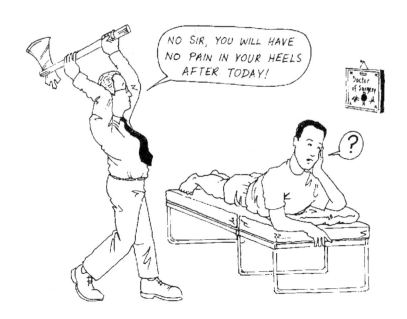

anyone with pronation, even those whose only exercise is a walk to the shops for the newspaper. It is a sprain or tear to the posterior tibial muscle (8). This originates in the back of your lower leg bone and literally holds your arches up. The cause of true shin splints is that pronation or rolling of the foot literally tugs the posterior tibial muscle away from the tibia bone. This progresses and worsens over time. Properly made orthotics are an absolute must and will clear-up shin splint. Accuracy in capturing the non-weight-bearing arch must be strongly emphasised.

It was his weakness – Achilles problems

Achilles problems present in many "shapes and sizes" and accurate diagnosis needs to be carried out to assess the type of problem involved. Many Achilles cases where minor injuries are annoyingly frequent should be assessed for biomechanical instability of the foot.

Excessive pronation or rolling at the rear foot may cause a constant strain on an Achilles tendon and pull it into a bow shape when viewed from the rear. This should be assessed and the appropriate orthotic prescribed to straighten the offending "bowing" and release the constant strain.

Ankle Symptoms

The ankle pain I am generally called upon to treat is caused by pronation (or fallen arches).

The ankle pain can take the form of one or both ankles being affected under the *malleolus*, the inner (medial) side being caused by a stretching of the tendons/ligaments, and the outer ankle area being caused by a "crushing" action.

If we treat this by correctly re-aligning the feet, we can save many years of pain

Severs Disease – see pages 63/64

Capsulitis (symptoms at the base of toes)

This affects the base of the toes where they join the metatarsals. The capsule/soft tissue area becomes inflamed. The causative factor can be hammer toes. The role of orthotics is to re-align the metatarsals and decrease pressure to this area.

Plantar fibromas ("lumps" under the arch)

These consist of harmless (but painful) tumours growing on the arch of the foot. The causative factor is not generally known but it is my educated guess that these occur as a result of an arch pulled tense by faulty foot positioning. Occasionally, these disappear on their own but, in my experience, they generally do not.

My orthotic approach is to take away the strain on the arch accurately and add special accommodations to keep the fibromas from being "crushed" underfoot. I have even used specially-drilled accommodations to the shell of the orthotic in a few extreme cases.

In rare cases, fibromas can be removed surgically but orthotics will still be needed to prevent recurrence.

Mid-foot arthritis

Flattened or hypermobile feet can give rise to "wear and tear" of the mid-foot's joints, wearing away the protective cartilage layers at the joints themselves, causing friction and wearing.

Affected patients can notice a painful grinding sensation in the feet, achiness and, of course, pain.

It is rare that mid-foot arthritis is not caused by faulty foot posture and my own approach is to re-align the feet with correct orthotics and a nutritional programme to counter the swelling and pain.

Osteoarthritis of the ankle

Osteoarthritis is literally wear and tear to a joint and the ankle is very prone to this, being the weight bearer that it is.

There is a slow deterioration of the cartilage at the joint caused either by an old injury or just by natural breaking down of the cartilage. The ankle is a large joint and so this can be especially disabling.

There is no cure for this arthritis, but the favoured procedure is re-alignment to the area by orthotics and nutritional and/or drug therapy to ease the inflammatory process. Sometimes ankle braces or supportive boots can assist the orthotic in the correction of the feet.

Surgery can also be offered to very severe cases by fusing the ankle joint so it is rigid and immovable.

CHAPTER NINE

THE IMPORTANCE OF PROPER
ORTHOTICS

As readers will have gathered by now, orthotics are a great love of mine, having saved me from a lifetime of pain and inactivity due to *Plantar Fasciitis* and shin splints. I thank God every time I run my usual ten miles (or spend hours at the gym) that I discovered the most incredible orthotics suited one hundred per cent to my individual needs, and I remember how I used to suffer sharp pain every time I walked, stood up or hobbled around on waking.

From a practitioner and prescriber's point of view, it gives immense pleasure to see patients derive such great benefits from our prescription orthotics, and to receive their thank you letters almost daily still gives me a great thrill and sense of pride. I think all practitioners should feel this, and any doctor or medical person who has lost this should find a new vocation.

One must consider all the alternatives when viewing a patient's condition and should not get tunnel vision that orthotics or indeed any other practice or discipline can be a cure-all. Biomechanical foot problems can only truly be countered by mechanical means, e.g. returning them to a normal stance. Occasionally one requires a wise mixture of surgery or treatment and orthotics to ensure a successful outcome, but in ninety-nine per cent of cases orthotics alone will suffice, perhaps with a little physical therapy.

The term "orthoses" comes from the word "orthos" meaning straight. It is normal thinking amongst most practitioners that a rigid orthotic is the ultimate. I have great argument with this and consider from vast experience of replacing rigid orthotics for patients who have got little or no benefit, or in some instances reacted adversely, that total rigidity in an orthotic is unnecessary. The human foot is designed to move within its limits and even though one corrects the biomechanical fault, it is by design that the orthotic should allow a little movement to remain. It has been shown time and time again that people who live outdoors with bare feet from a young age rarely, if ever, suffer biomechanical foot problems as all the muscles in the feet are going through a constant "workout". My own experience of this first hand was many years ago working with a Thai boxing (or Muay

Thai) team. I was osteopath for the team (as well as a fighter at that time) and had the great good fortune to be able to observe the feet of this great group of ladies and gents. Bearing in mind that most of these fighters trained for six to eight hours daily in bare feet and all were aged around 18-25, it was interesting to note that their individual foot posture was near perfect.

When we observe traditional Thai boxing training we see that all of it is done balanced on the balls of the feet. So it necessarily follows that all the musculature around the ankles, lower legs and throughout the feet is constantly engaged in pure strength training. In consequence of the above, the feet, with their constant gruelling exercise programme, were able to maintain a perfect posture.

One of those fighters continued as a great friend of mine - long after his active fighting days. It was most interesting to note that within six months of ceasing barefoot training six hours a day, his feet had dropped into pronation followed by a pattern of pronatory pains, for which we prescribed orthotics successfully.

The above story illustrates what can be done to strengthen feet from an early age, but for ninety-nine per cent of patients a Muay Thai training school or a Zola Budd running programme is out of the equation!

Many exercises, such as picking up pencils with the toes or rolling the ankles, are given to patients with pronation and dropped medial arches. This approach is akin to carrying out a ten minute gym workout daily and expecting a musculature like that of Arnold Schwarzenegger. The Thai boxing story clearly illustrates the amount of work needed to build foot muscles strong enough to almost "take over" from the lax or overstretched ligaments and support the bodies weight. This would be like expecting to lift a hundred kilos with one bicep muscle.

In view of all this, in a practical normal life we need orthotics to do sixty per cent of the job of the foot's intrinsic strength. To return to the point I was making earlier, the reader will have gathered that the perfect foot has a natural amount of "bounce" or movement and is not to be held solidly, but encouraged to stay "firmly" in its desired position of talar neutral, allowing the foot to flex slightly with the orthotic.

At the other end of the spectrum from hard unforgiving orthotic materials, we do not expect major results from a pad-type device. In other words soft orthotics should be discouraged as these prove to be little more than a padding instrument merely adding a squishy layer under the foot. The added problem with these is that they take up a lot of the available room in the shoe and limit footwear choice. As a stalwart advocate of correct orthotic devices, I only ever consider these orthotic pads as a temporary measure.

As a clinic, we are constantly appalled at the quality of so-called orthotics worn by patients who come to us, (these having been prescribed by previous practitioners). Most are rigid, but the models that irritate me the most are the off-the-shelf shells with postings stuck on to emulate a prescription device. The mere fact that the arch bears no resemblance at all to the patient's non-weight-bearing foot is immediate evidence of its unsuitability, without the addition of these superfluous paddings and postings that simply cannot add accuracy, as the body of the orthotic is already seriously faulty.

Built on years of observation, my philosophy is that any orthotic that is not specifically designed for your individual foot and all its nuances should never be worn. My reasoning is that one may, if very lucky, adjust the pain of the presenting problem, but the cost to other areas of the musculoskeletal system can be high. I make no apologies for repeating this. I want my readers to absorb this thoroughly.

An imperfect foot will cause unnecessary wear and tear, and strain to the foot, ankles, knees, hips and lower back. To push the foot from one faulty position to another by using off-the-shelf devices is asking for future problems.

Do not be confused by this text as many "accommodative" devices may be useful; for example, a shielding device for painful bunions or an implement to part the toes and protect against a painful corn. These have a positive place as they do not interfere with Mother Nature's delicate biomechanical balance. At the same time I do like to see, where possible, the causative factor dealt with at the same time as using an accommodative device.

The correct type of orthotic material used is a major factor particularly in dealing with *plantar fasciitis* or problems emanating from the plantar aspect of the foot. Daily, we witness people who consult us with orthotics that bring too much pressure to bear against the *plantar aponeurosis*, which is already inflamed and torn. The orthotic should be able to "give" slightly in its structure particularly under the *aponeurosis*. With this in mind the orthotic has to support the foot effectively, which means that a mere soft orthotic will be unsuitable.

The ideal orthotic employs a memory shell that will move with the patient's weight and foot type and can be counted on not to lose shape over the years.

When using these materials it is even possible to employ a 1mm gauge material, accurately padded in crucial areas, to give support with inbuilt pertinent flexibility.

A practitioner dealing with orthotics should have a great deal of experience in the use of functional foot orthotics. They should be able to explain fully why an orthotic is needed in the first place, and be fully conversant with any further options such as surgery or manual treatment. But of utmost importance is the correct knowledge of what steps to take should the orthotic be either painful or not working, for example knowing when to add height to arches (or to lower them), if and when to add or change rear or forefoot support or adjust padding etc.

An orthotic laboratory will do most of the work when an orthotic is needed, but it never ceases to amaze us how many practitioners are completely lost when it comes to adjustments. In short, always find a practitioner with a high level of experience and skills.

"Starter" orthotics

I gave much thought to the process of foot adaptation to orthotic correction, and came up with an answer that has assisted many people to adapt to orthotics.

The problem lies in the fact that it is often difficult for patients with rigid arches and/or badly pronated rear feet (ankles) to cope with a full correction from the beginning.

So I developed a system of what I term "starter" orthotics, whereby I prescribe a lower and more flexible arch and a lesser rear-foot correction. In cases of patients where the rear foot has had time to "solidify" into the pronated position and the arch fascias have become "fibrous", these "starters" have proved themselves very effective through many years of prescription.

In extreme cases, I have been known to correct the feet in three moves, using two "starter" models of gradually-heightening arches and rearfoot correction.

This simply allows the feet time to adapt to each stage of correction without forcing the foot to change in one correction, which can cause much discomfort.

Coupled with the work I have done on arch movement, this has been an overall success, proven over many years.

How long do orthotics take to work?

This is a golden question and one which has no definitive answer.

I have found my own patients differ greatly but, because of the implementation of my work with arch movement, we tend towards a much faster resolution with around 80% of people out of pain within days. 10% will take a few weeks or months to heal, and the remaining 10% may need any number of adjustments.

Adjustments - the best-kept secret in orthotics

I am always surprised how little prescribers of orthotics know about the vital role which adjustments play in orthotic prescription.

Certain patients may need the assistance of the prescriber to help them adapt to the orthotic. There can be many possible reasons for this; for example the patient may not cope with their "perfect" arch height, rear or forefoot correction and even prescription paddings.

The prescriber must be aware of what to do in these cases as this is a critical part of orthotic prescribing, and one that is all too often poorly understood by prescribers who find this all very confusing. One may need to lead the patient through several adjustments to reach that goal, and knowing how to carry this out at every stage is vital.

I generally do around one or two adjustments on 10% of patients but higher numbers are not uncommon with difficult cases needing perhaps four to five. (My "record" was for a lady with an incredibly complex and extreme *pes cavus* foot, where I performed seventeen adjustments before she was completely out of pain. (Luckily this was a one-off.)

The reason for multiple adjustments, thankfully rare, is that each adjustment has to be "trialled" by the patient to see where, and indeed if, we need to go with the next one. I will admit this can be a complex study that has been accurately described as "half art, half science" but is a topic in which the prescriber needs many years' experience in order to perfect its modalities.

Speeding the healing process

The body is an incredibly complex machine that requires correct nutrition to heal and function.

There are several natural "anti-inflammatories" that I prescribe, all aimed at not just hiding problems but greatly assisting the repair process.

My favourites are generally certain nutritional products and occasionally herbal supplements. The skill with these is to tailor them to the individual patient and to source the highest quality possible.

I have used this approach for quite some time now and found the results highly favourable, speeding up healing and lowering pain levels far quicker.

I am not against conventional drug therapy as many lives would be lost without it, but I have found that pharmaceutical drugs never offer great results in plantar fasciitis or metatarsal cases.

Like drug therapy, the natural approach can only work once the biomechanical positioning (the "cause") has been corrected.

My favourites are individual combinations of <u>high quality</u> products such as Bromelain, turmeric, omega 3, devils claw, cats claw, arnica gels/mother tinctures, glucosamine and similar safe and effective products.

However, like anything in life, quality is paramount as there are cheaper, less effective versions on the market.

SUMMARY

Each of your feet is a complex tool, capable of great feats of engineering – carrying your frame wherever and whenever you wish to transport yourself somewhere. They slavishly follow instructions from the brain and nervous system, never-ending in their obedience to the user who pushes them thousands of times every day.

When walking, every step carries two-and-a-half times our body weight right through the core of the foot. In the case of a runner one can only guess at the weight ratio per kilo of body weight per foot.

Is it really any wonder that these miracles of nature get biomechanical problems? I have only covered a fraction of the vast list of conditions associated with feet, and then only from a biomechanical point of view. I have stressed that this is a volume for the layman, but I can thoroughly recommend any of the books I have used as references for your further perusal.

Your feet should receive your every care and attention, and when things go wrong only consult the very "cream" of practitioners, use the correct orthotics and if it seems like nothing is helping, keep looking and trying new and better modalities and specialists.

Take the greatest care of yourself and your feet and I thank you sincerely for finding the time in your busy life to read my humble volume.

God bless.

Les Bailey, PhD.
Senior Biomechanics Consultant

<u>Contact Me</u>
Should you wish to contact me with any questions, or for orthotic enquiries, please e-mail:
drlesbailey@yahoo.co.uk

For consultations/general enquiries contact:
<u>The Clinic</u>
0845 520 1950
www.thecliniconline.co.uk

OTHER RECOMMENDED READING

The Clinician's Guide to Plantar Fasciitis; Les Bailey, PhD.,
Currently being written, this book is the professionals' guide to foot and heel pain.

It is aimed at doctors, podiatrists, physiotherapists, osteopaths and chiropractors.

REFERENCES

1. Ranowat & Positano, *Disorders of the Heel, Rearfoot and Ankle* (1st edition), Churchill Livingstone, 1999. ISBN 0-443-07838-6.

2. Tontora and Grabowski, *Principles of Anatomy and Physiology* (9th edition), John Wiley & Sons Inc, 2000. ISBN 0-471-36692-7.

3. Gray's Anatomy (31st edition), Longmans, 1954.

4. *Dynamic Loading of the Plantar Aponeurosis in Walking* Erdemir *et al*, 86 (3) 546.

5. www.arthroscopy.com/sp09001.htm

6. Dr William Rossi, *The Arches and Some Controversial Views*. www.unshod.org/pfbc/pfrossi.htm

7. *The Treatment of 100 Common Diseases by New Acupuncture*, Hong Kong: Medicine & Health Publishing Co, 1988.

8. William Southmayd M.D. and Marshall Hoffman, *Sports Health*, Perigee, 1984. ISBN 0-399-51107-5